Fast Facts for Healthcare Professionals

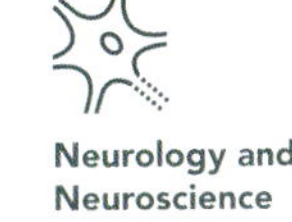

Neurology and Neuroscience

Excessive Daytime Sleepiness Associated with Obstructive Sleep Apnea

Walter T McNicholas MD FRCPI FERS
Department of Respiratory and Sleep Medicine
St Vincent's Hospital Group
University College Dublin
Dublin, Ireland

Ulf Kallweit MD FEAN
Clinical Sleep and Neuroimmunology
Institute for Immunology and Center for Biomedical Education and Research
University of Witten/Herdecke
Witten, Germany

Gert Jan Lammers MD PhD FEAN
Department of Neurology
Leiden University Medical Center, Leiden, and
Sleep-Wake Center SEIN
Heemstede, The Netherlands

Joerg Steier MD PhD FRCP
Lane Fox Unit/Sleep Disorders Centre
Guy's and St Thomas' NHS Foundation Trust and
Centre for Human & Applied Physiological Sciences
King's College London
London, UK

Declaration of Independence
This book is as balanced and practical as we can make it.
Ideas for improvement are always welcome: fastfacts@karger.com

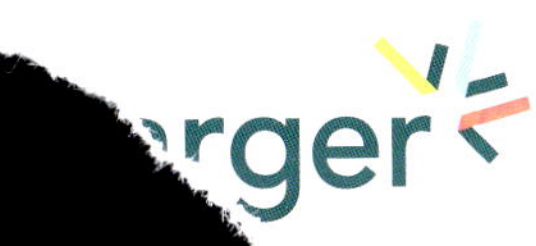

HEALTHCARE

Fast Facts: Excessive Daytime Sleepiness Associated with Obstructive Sleep Apnea
First published 2022

S. Karger Publishers Ltd, Elizabeth House, Queen Street, Abingdon,
Oxford OX14 3LN, UK; tel: +44 (0)1235 523233

Book orders can be placed by telephone or email, or via the website.
Please telephone +41 61 306 1440 or email orders@karger.com
To order via the website, please go to karger.com

A CIP record for this title is available from the British Library.

ISBN 978-3-318-02379-4

McNicholas WT (Walter)
Fast Facts: Excessive Daytime Sleepiness Associated with Obstructive Sleep Apnea/
Walter T McNicholas, Ulf Kallweit, Gert Jan Lammers, Joerg Steier

Typesetting by Amnet, Chennai, India; printed in the UK with Xpedient Print.

An independent publication developed by S. Karger Publishers Ltd and provided as a service to medicine. Jazz Pharmaceuticals has provided sponsorship for the production of this book. This publication has been initiated by S. Karger Publishers Ltd with no inp[illegible] from Jazz Pharmaceuticals for the subject, selection of authors and no editorial in[illegible] any way other than a review for technical accuracy.

List of abbreviations

AHI: apnea–hypopnea index

CPAP: continuous positive airway pressure

DVLA: Driver and Vehicle Licensing Agency (UK)

EDS: excessive daytime sleepiness

EMA: European Medicines Agency

ENS: excessive need for sleep

ESS: Epworth Sleepiness Scale

ICSD-3: International Classification of Sleep Disorders, 3rd edition

MAD: mandibular advancement device

MSLT: Multiple Sleep Latency Test

MWT: Maintenance of Wakefulness Test

OSA: obstructive sleep apnea

OSAS: obstructive sleep apnea syndrome

PAP: positive airway pressure

REM: rapid-eye-movement (sleep)

SAT: Sleep Apnoea Trust

Introduction

Independently, excessive daytime sleepiness (EDS) and obstructive sleep apnea (OSA) are both highly prevalent in the general population. OSA is the type of sleep-disordered breathing that most often causes EDS.

EDS is a multifaceted complaint that usually involves disabling symptoms such as an increased need for sleep, impaired sustained attention, automatic behavior (behaviors that are performed without conscious knowledge or full voluntary control), cognitive complaints (especially those linked to poor memory) and sometimes sleep inertia. Lack of awareness and failure to recognize the severity of the effects of these symptoms on quality of life often leads to under- or delayed diagnosis, which prevents patients from receiving adequate treatment, and also prevents referral from primary care.

Despite EDS being a common complaint, best practice regarding the management of patients with OSA is not well defined because no evidence-based guidelines are available. This first edition of *Fast Facts: Excessive Daytime Sleepiness Associated with Obstructive Sleep Apnea* discusses the difficulties in formulating a definition of EDS that appropriately considers the experiences and features of daytime sleepiness, as well as the need for improved guidance regarding clinical practice. Up-to-date information is provided for the accurate assessment of EDS in patients with OSA with a focus on persisting complaints of EDS after standard treatment, alongside a discussion of best practice in terms of their management and support. This handbook will be of use to people working across the healthcare spectrum.

Neurology and Neuroscience

1 Epidemiology and etiology

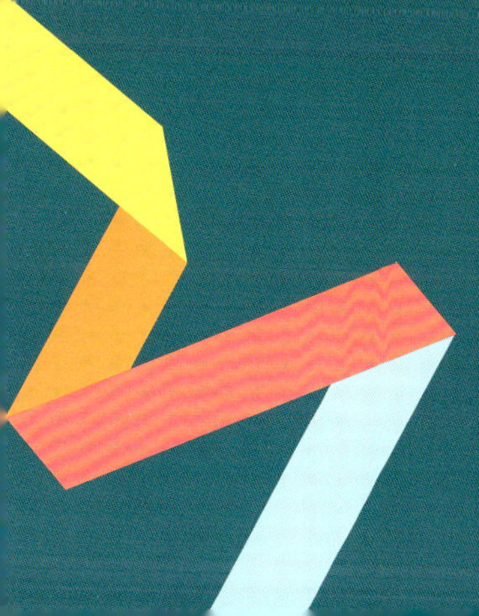

HEALTHCARE

Definitions

Obstructive sleep apnea (OSA) is highly prevalent, but its epidemiology must be considered at two levels. The first (and broadest) level is the prevalence of the disorder when defined only as the frequency of obstructive breathing events during sleep, usually expressed as the frequency of apneas and hypopneas per hour of sleep: the apnea–hypopnea index (AHI). Apnea reflects complete cessation, whereas hypopnea reflects reduced breathing with associated oxygen desaturation and/or arousal. The second (more restricted) level is when OSA is defined as a clinical syndrome where the AHI is combined with compatible clinical symptoms, most notably excessive daytime sleepiness (EDS), when it is often referred to as obstructive sleep apnea syndrome (OSAS) or, less commonly, obstructive sleep apnea–hypopnea syndrome. However, there is no universally accepted terminology to describe the syndrome, which is frequently referred to in the literature as OSA, with some authors referring to OSA expressed only in terms of the AHI as sleep-disordered breathing.

An important factor to consider regarding the definition of OSAS is the poor correlation between the AHI and symptoms such as EDS,[1] which compromises the establishment of clear-cut criteria for the definition of the clinical syndrome. This is evident from reports that have found EDS to be a common manifestation in population studies of OSA prevalence, even among participants with an AHI less than 5 per hour.[2] These considerations have prompted the re-evaluation of the AHI's clinical value in the assessment of clinical significance and a search for variables that may be more effective, especially in the prediction of comorbidity. Efforts are also being made to improve the clinical prediction of significant OSA in different populations by evaluating different phenotypic clusters that include traits such as sex, body mass index, symptoms and comorbidities. A joint working group of the European Respiratory Society and European Sleep Research Society recently proposed a classification system that enables supplementary grading of OSA severity based on symptoms and comorbidity, which may improve the identification of clinically significant OSA and facilitate improved treatment planning.[3]

Epidemiology

OSA, expressed only in terms of the AHI, is estimated to affect up to one billion people worldwide,[4] and population studies from North America, Europe and Australasia have indicated prevalence figures of up to 50% in adults (Figure 1.1). Indeed, one general population study from Switzerland reported an AHI greater than 15 per hour in almost 50% of men, although the prevalence of AHI greater than 15 per hour combined with symptoms (OSAS) in the same population was less than 10% (Figure 1.2).[5]

EDS as an independent manifestation is also highly prevalent and was recently reported to affect around 20% of the normal adult population.[6] It is frequently lifestyle induced, with contributory factors such as poor sleep hygiene and inadequate sleep duration. Despite OSA being the medical disorder most often associated with EDS, EDS has been reported to be more common in women and in participants reporting insomnia.[6]

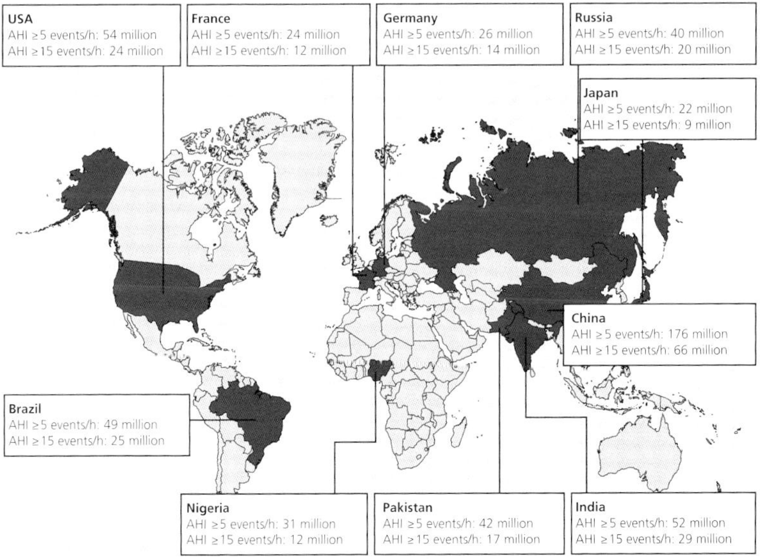

Figure 1.1 Estimation of the global prevalence of OSA. Reproduced with permission from Benjafield et al., 2019.[4]

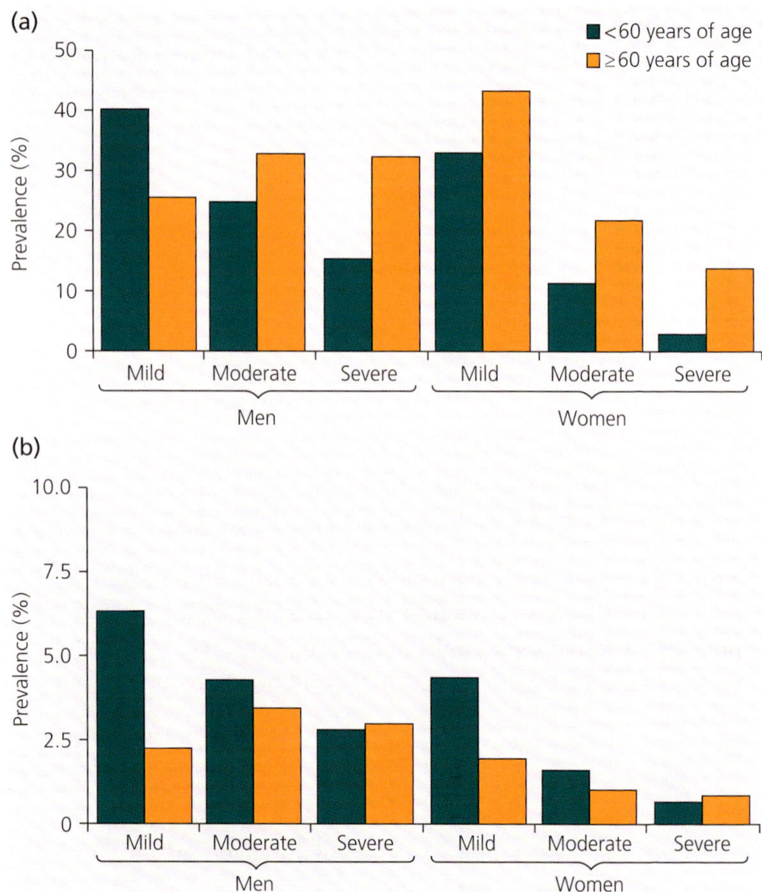

Figure 1.2 Prevalence of (a) sleep-disordered breathing and (b) OSAS by age and sex. Reproduced with permission from Heinzer et al., 2015.[5]

Sex differences. OSA is more common in men than women, with a ratio of around 2:1 in general population studies (see Figure 1.2).[5] The ratio is often higher in sleep clinic populations, which may relate to differences in symptom profiles that prompt men to seek medical attention earlier than women.

Age. OSA is more common in the elderly, who tend to be less symptomatic, and thus the clinical significance of OSA in the elderly is uncertain.[7] The prevalence in children is much lower than that in adults,[8] and a lower AHI threshold than that applied to adults is considered clinically significant (≥1 per hour for children compared with ≥5 per hour for adults). The prevalence of OSA has been steadily increasing over recent decades, which likely reflects the rising global incidence of obesity.

Genetic factors are increasingly recognised to play an important role in the development of OSAS. Prevalence in first-degree relatives of patients with OSAS is about two-fold higher than that found in first-degree relatives of healthy controls,[9] and the likelihood of OSAS increases with the number of affected relatives. Potential genetic factors include upper airway morphology, body fat distribution and the control of breathing abnormalities.[10] Ethnic factors may also play a role, with craniofacial structure being an important risk factor in people from East Asia.

Comorbidities. The prevalence of OSA in patients with cardiovascular and metabolic diseases is significantly higher than in the general population. A recent report indicated this to be especially so for hypertensive patients with a nocturnal non-dipping blood pressure profile.[11]

Etiology

The fundamental basis of OSA is a recurring obstruction of the oropharyngeal airway during sleep. The maintenance of a patent upper airway requires the collapsing forces applied during inspiration and the counteracting actions of dilating muscles, especially the genioglossus, to be balanced.[12] Narrowing of the upper airway increases the collapsing forces (Figure 1.3). The Mallampati score, which is commonly used in anesthetic practice to evaluate upper airway caliber, is widely used to assess the extent of narrowing of the oropharynx in a clinical setting. A score of 3 or 4 is typical in patients with OSA. Oropharyngeal narrowing is believed to be influenced by a combination of factors.

Genetic factors include craniofacial abnormalities, especially those associated with micro- or retrognathia such as Pierre Robin and Treacher Collins syndromes. Adenotonsillar hypertrophy is

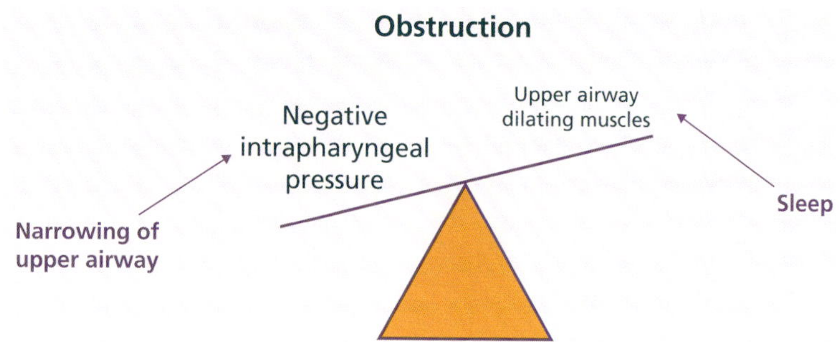

Figure 1.3 Mechanisms of upper airway obstruction in OSA.

a major factor contributing to airway narrowing in children with OSA.

Structural factors. Upper airway obstruction is most likely to occur during sleep because reduced tone and contractility of dilating muscles are normal features of sleep, especially during rapid-eye-movement (REM) sleep. Diminished neuromuscular responsiveness of the dilating muscles may be an important contributing factor in some patients and may involve local neuropathy in the upper airway. Obesity is also believed to contribute to narrowing of the oropharyngeal airway as a result of fat deposition in the neck.

Pathophysiological factors that have recently been suggested to be important contributors to the development of OSA are the arousal threshold and loop gain. A low arousal threshold adversely affects sleep stability, while a high loop gain promotes respiratory control instability, and both factors indirectly increase upper airway collapsibility. Abnormalities in the arousal threshold and/or loop gain have been identified in at least one-third of patients with OSA.[13] The recognition of different pathophysiological traits may improve treatment choices for individual patients, which is especially important as increasing attention is given to potential pharmacological targets that may replace, or supplement, traditional therapies such as continuous positive airway pressure (CPAP).

Key points – epidemiology and etiology

- OSA, defined only as the AHI, is estimated to affect up to one billion people worldwide.
- The definition of a clinically significant OSAS is made difficult by the poor correlation between the AHI and symptoms such as EDS.
- The prevalence in men is twice that of women, but women tend to be underrepresented in clinic-based samples.
- OSA is also common in children and adenotonsillar hypertrophy is the most common etiology.
- The most important etiologic factor in OSA is narrowing of the oropharyngeal airway and genetic factors play an important role.
- The arousal threshold and loop gain are additional etiologic factors that may open new avenues for therapy.

References

1. Deegan PC, McNicholas WT. Predictive value of clinical features for the obstructive sleep apnoea syndrome. *Eur Resp J* 1996;9:117–24.
2. Gottlieb DJ, Whitney CW, Bonekat WH et al. Relation of sleepiness to respiratory disturbance index: the Sleep Heart Health Study. *Am J Respir Crit Care Med* 1999;159:502–7.
3. Randerath W, Bassetti CL, Bonsignore MR et al. Challenges and perspectives in obstructive sleep apnoea: report by an *ad hoc* working group of the Sleep Disordered Breathing Group of the European Respiratory Society and the European Sleep Research Society. *Eur Resp J* 2018;52:1702616.
4. Benjafield AV, Ayas NT, Eastwood PR et al. Estimation of the global prevalence and burden of obstructive sleep apnoea: a literature-based analysis. *Lancet Respir Med* 2019;7:687–98.
5. Heinzer R, Vat S, Marques-Vidal P et al. Prevalence of sleep-disordered breathing in the general population: the HypnoLaus study. *Lancet Respir Med* 2015;3:310–18.
6. Kolla BP, He JP, Mansukhani MP et al. Excessive sleepiness and associated symptoms in the U.S. adult population: prevalence, correlates, and comorbidity. *Sleep Health* 2020;6:79–87.

7. Sforza E, Roche F, Thomas-Anterion C et al. Cognitive function and sleep related breathing disorders in a healthy elderly population: the SYNAPSE study. *Sleep* 2010;33:515–21.
8. Marcus CL, Brooks LJ, Draper KA et al. Diagnosis and management of childhood obstructive sleep apnea syndrome. *Pediatrics* 2012;130:576–84.
9. Gislason T, Johannsson JH, Haraldsson A et al. Familial predisposition and cosegregation analysis of adult obstructive sleep apnea and the sudden infant death syndrome. *Am J Respir Crit Care Med* 2002;166:833–8.
10. Kent BD, Ryan S, McNicholas WT. The genetics of obstructive sleep apnoea. *Curr Opin Pulm Med* 2010;16:536–42.
11. Crinion SJ, Ryan S, Kleinerova J et al. Nondipping nocturnal blood pressure predicts sleep apnea in patients with hypertension. *J Clin Sleep Med* 2019;15:957–63.
12. Deegan PC, McNicholas WT. Pathophysiology of obstructive sleep apnoea. *Eur Resp J* 1995; 8:1161–78.
13. Eckert DJ, White DP, Jordan AS et al. Defining phenotypic causes of obstructive sleep apnea. Identification of novel therapeutic targets. *Am J Respir Crit Care Med* 2013;188:996–1004.

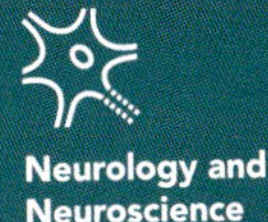

2 Clinical features and diagnosis

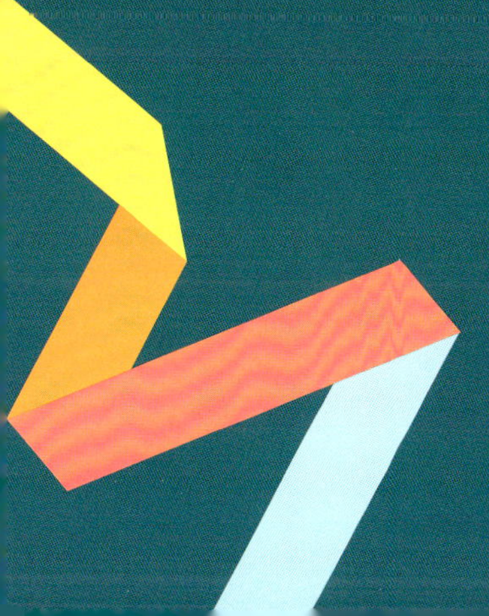

HEALTHCARE

What is excessive daytime sleepiness?

During normal daytime hours, healthy adults with a normal sleep–wake rhythm are generally expected to stay awake, even in monotonous situations. Accordingly, EDS can be defined as sleepiness and/or sleep occurring during the daytime in a situation when an individual would normally desire and be expected to stay awake. Formulating a definition of EDS that also appropriately appreciates the experiences and features of daytime sleepiness is difficult.

The International Classification of Sleep Disorders, 3rd edition (ICSD-3),[1] uses a definition of EDS that is limited to sleep-related features: 'daily episodes of an irrepressible need to sleep or daytime lapses into sleep', which occur for at least 3 months.

Although this definition is workable, it does not acknowledge that EDS is a multifaceted complaint that usually involves disabling symptoms such as impaired sustained attention, automatic behavior (behaviors that are performed without conscious knowledge or full voluntary control), cognitive complaints (especially those linked to poor memory) and sometimes sleep inertia. Failure to recognise the severity of the effects of these symptoms on quality of life leads to underdiagnosis preventing adequate treatment, and also limits referral from primary care.

Differentiation from tiredness and fatigue. EDS is a symptom and not a diagnosis, and is not even necessarily a symptom of a sleep or breathing disorder; lifestyle and external factors leading to sleep deprivation and/or disruption may, for example, induce sleepiness that is perceived to be 'excessive'. For correct interpretation and workup, it is important to separate EDS from tiredness and fatigue, which are qualitatively different complaints.

Tiredness is partial or complete depletion of energy or strength after exercise.

Fatigue can be defined as physical and/or mental exhaustion, with difficulty initiating or sustaining voluntary activity, thus limiting an individual's ability to work and/or quality of life. Increased rest or sleep does not necessarily improve fatigue.

Assessment. The complex, multifaceted nature of sleepiness is reflected by the potentially discordant subjective and objective findings that can be obtained when assessing it. For example, those who report daytime sleepiness may or may not fulfill criteria for the Multiple Sleep Latency Test (MSLT), which is considered to be an objective test for the assessment and quantification of EDS. Conversely, people who have an MSLT result that indicates daytime sleepiness may not always have a complaint of sleepiness.

Phenotypes. Two different phenotypes of EDS are described: one that is characterized by an inability to remain awake during the day without a relevant increase of sleep over a 24-hour period, and the other by an increased amount of sleep rather than an inability to remain awake. A group of European experts recently suggested the following criteria for both phenotypes of EDS, acknowledging the multifaceted nature of the complaint.[2]

Excessive daytime sleepiness (EDS). EDS is often accompanied by cognitive difficulties (particularly memory complaints) and emotional difficulties, including irritability and distractibility, and headache. The criteria for the presence of EDS are:

- daily presence of a feeling of daytime sleepiness throughout most of the day as opposed to symptoms of fatigue
- daily or near-daily inability to stay awake in monotonous situations with unintended napping and possibly sleep attacks
- at least one of the following: an acquired need for scheduled napping during the day, difficulty with sustained attention and vigilance, and automatic behaviors that can be attributed to EDS.

Excessive need for sleep (ENS). The criteria for ENS are the daily or near-daily presence of all the following clinical symptoms and complaints:

- an increased need for sleep in normal daily life, which comprises at least 10 hours of sleep per 24 hours and/or at least 9 hours of nocturnal sleep
- the presence of at least one of the symptoms of EDS listed above and/or the presence of sleep inertia/sleep drunkenness
- sleep extension not (fully) eliminating the previously listed symptoms and complaints.

Diagnosis

History taking. The patient's complaint should be the starting point. Many patients, although experiencing sleepiness, express their complaint as 'I feel so tired'; therefore, primary care providers must always verify exactly what the patient means. If sleepiness is meant, the second aspect that needs to be clarified is whether the patient has an inability to stay awake or an increased need for sleep. The impact on daily functioning should also be assessed. People may have combinations of EDS, ENS and/or fatigue. Coexisting fatigue may even exaggerate the burden of EDS because most people suffer less from EDS when they are active; EDS complaints typically increase during monotonous activities and inactivity, and improve or even disappear when the person is being active (similar to the experience of healthy people when they are sleep-deprived).

Whether a complaint of EDS is behaviorally induced or caused by a disorder is not always easily determined for two main reasons. First, there is no qualitative difference between EDS complaints induced by chronic sleep deprivation and complaints caused by a disorder. Second, there are large, inborn interindividual differences in need for sleep that prevent primary care providers from drawing conclusions based on absolute durations/amounts of (nocturnal) sleep. Some people do not need more than 7 hours of sleep per day, while others need 8 hours or more to prevent EDS.

Sleep schedules. Because the most frequent cause of EDS is chronic sleep deprivation induced by sleep curtailment and/or a severely disturbed sleep–wake rhythm, it is essential that sleep schedules are asked about during history taking (see Subjective tests and questionnaires on page 23). The use of sleep diaries and actigraphy can identify such disturbance (see Objective tests for sleep on page 24). When sleep deprivation is the probable cause, but also in cases of doubt, sleep extension should be advised and monitored for success. Having considerably longer (nocturnal) sleep times during weekends and holidays is an indirect indication of chronic sleep deprivation and ENS. Another clue may be the temporal relationship between the onset of EDS and a change in sleep duration and/or schedule. Advice regarding sleep extension should be based on the amount of sleep before the complaints started and the current time spent in bed for nocturnal sleep. The advice will almost always be to stay in bed for at least 7.5 hours, often longer.

Increased need for sleep must be separated from an inborn, but not pathological, need for sleep. In people with a naturally large need for sleep, the sleepiness complaint typically occurs when sleep is curtailed, and disappears when sleep duration is extended. A large need for sleep must also be separated from long periods spent in bed (called clinophilia), which is mainly seen in patients with psychiatric disorders.

Circadian problems may also cause EDS complaints. For example, people suffering from (severe) delayed sleep phase syndrome may have difficulty initiating nocturnal sleep early enough to allow them to fulfill their sleep needs when they are forced to rise early in the morning to care for children or fulfill work obligations. History taking can usually aid identification: they typically have difficulty rising in the morning and may feel sleepy during the day, but start to feel better again in the evening. Circadian disorders and sleep curtailment that is entirely behaviorally induced cannot always be separated, but increased nocturnal sleep duration should be the aim for both populations.

Elderly people who are healthy are not sleepier than younger people. However, inactivity, which may or may not be induced by comorbidity, may impact existing EDS complaints.

Medication that may cause daytime sleepiness. Several medications may induce daytime sleepiness. Various mechanisms may be involved: a direct daytime sedative effect, a direct effect on nocturnal sleep and/or an indirect effect through inducing sleep-related apneas (Table 2.1). Most substances directly influence neurotransmitter systems in the brain that are involved in the regulation of sleep and wakefulness.

Assessment of excessive sleepiness. Similar to history taking, ancillary investigations, including tests such as the MSLT, cannot reliably differentiate between EDS complaints induced by lifestyle problems and those induced by a real sleep disorder. This makes interpretation of ancillary investigations complex and highly dependent on the context, particularly the presence of sleep deprivation. Unfortunately, there are no biomarkers that can reliably differentiate between the two.

TABLE 2.1

Substances that may cause daytime sleepiness*

Examples of frequently used substances, or classes of drugs, that may directly cause EDS[3]

- Sedatives: benzodiazepines, γ-aminobutyric acid agonists, antihistaminergic substances, anticholinergics
- Certain anticonvulsant drugs: particularly barbiturates, but also non-barbiturates mainly when initiating treatment or when overdosed; carbamazepine is a well-known example
- Opiates: particularly when initiating treatment; not much is known about chronic use
- Neuroleptics and sedative antidepressants
- Occasionally dopamine agonists

Substances that may induce a disturbance of nocturnal sleep

- Alcohol: a sedative that facilitates sleep onset at night, but disturbs sleep maintenance; may also aggravate hypopneas and/or apneas
- β-Blockers
- β-Mimetics
- Steroids
- Stimulants
- Caffeine: a stimulant that may disturb nocturnal sleep, particularly when large amounts are consumed in the evening
- Smoking: nicotine is a stimulant

Substances that may have an indirect effect on nocturnal sleep

- Opiates: may induce or aggravate nocturnal hyponeas and/or apneas
- Alcohol: a sedative that facilitates sleep onset at night, but disturbs sleep maintenance; may also aggravate hypopneas and/or apneas
- Benzodiazepines and other γ-aminobutyric acid agonists may induce or aggravate hypopneas and/or apneas

*Only substances that are frequently used are listed.
Adapted from American Academy of Sleep Medicine, 2014[1] and Ruigt and van Gerven, 2018.[3]

As mentioned previously, it makes sense to conduct sleep registrations (including the MSLT) only after sleep deprivation has been excluded; in other words, if complaints remain after sleep extension. Ancillary investigations can focus on all aspects of EDS/ENS and it is best to use several approaches during the diagnostic process.

Subjective tests and questionnaires

The Epworth Sleepiness Scale. The most frequently used questionnaire is the Epworth Sleepiness Scale (ESS), which provides a score for sleep over the preceding weeks (Table 2.2).[4] The maximum score is 24 points and a score greater than 10 indicates an unusual level of tiredness.

The Stanford Sleepiness Scale is a short questionnaire that assesses momentary feelings of sleepiness. The participant is asked to rate their alertness at different times of the day on a scale of 1–7, where 1 indicates feeling active, alert and wide awake, and 7 indicates no longer fighting sleep, soon to fall asleep and dream-like thoughts.

TABLE 2.2

Questions in the ESS

In the following situations, how likely are you to doze off or fall asleep?

- Sitting and reading
- Watching TV
- Sitting, inactive in a public place (theatre, cinema, meeting etc.)
- In a car as a passenger for 1 hour with no break
- Sitting, talking to someone
- Sitting, quietly after lunch (no alcohol)
- Stopping for a few minutes in traffic while driving
- Lying down to rest in the afternoon when circumstances permit

People completing the ESS are asked to rate each item from 0–3, where 0 = would never fall asleep in that situation, 1 = a slight chance of falling asleep, 2 = a medium chance of falling asleep and 3 = a high chance of falling asleep in that situation. The scores are then added together. A total score ≥ 11 indicates an unusual level of sleepiness. Adapted from Johns, 1991.[4]

Objective tests for sleep

Actigraphy involves a small device worn on the wrist that can detect and quantify movement during sleep for up to several weeks. Results can then be visualized on an actogram (Figure 2.1); the concept is that people who are awake move almost constantly to some extent, while people who sleep quietly hardly move at all. Although movement is not generally a reliable way to assess sleep, the combination of actigraphy and sleep diary data provides a reliable and feasible way to objectify sleep–wake schedules, including time in bed. Actigraphy therefore plays an important role in detecting sleep curtailment and/or severely disturbed sleep–wake schedules as causes of EDS. It can also be used to verify whether patients' previously disturbed sleep–wake schedules have improved.

Polysomnography is the gold-standard test for measuring sleep. Electroencephalographic signals, eye movements and muscle tone are simultaneously registered, and the combined result defines the wake and various sleep stages. In addition, respiratory parameters, muscle activity in the legs and electrocardiogram data are recorded.

The Multiple Sleep Latency Test (MSLT) is considered by many to be the gold standard for objectifying EDS,[5] although it has been the subject of debate in recent years. The MSLT comprises an in-laboratory test that is performed after nocturnal polysomnography (mainly to document that there has been enough nocturnal sleep the night before the test, but also to document existing sleep disturbances or disorders), and polysomnography is used to assess the occurrence of sleep. Participants are asked to try to fall asleep while lying down on a bed in a quiet room with a dim light. There may be four or five sessions spread over the day of 20 minutes each, although they may last longer when the participants fall asleep to allow for the occurrence of sleep-onset REM sleep. The primary outcome measure is the average of all sleep-onset latencies; when no sleep occurs, sleep latency is noted as 20 minutes. A secondary outcome measure is the occurrence of sleep-onset REM episodes.

The Maintenance of Wakefulness Test (MWT), in contrast to the MSLT, comprises a test in which participants are asked to stay awake and sleep is measured.[5] Polysomnography of the preceding night is not required, but polysomnographic techniques are used to assess the occurrence of sleep. Participants are instructed to sit still and remain

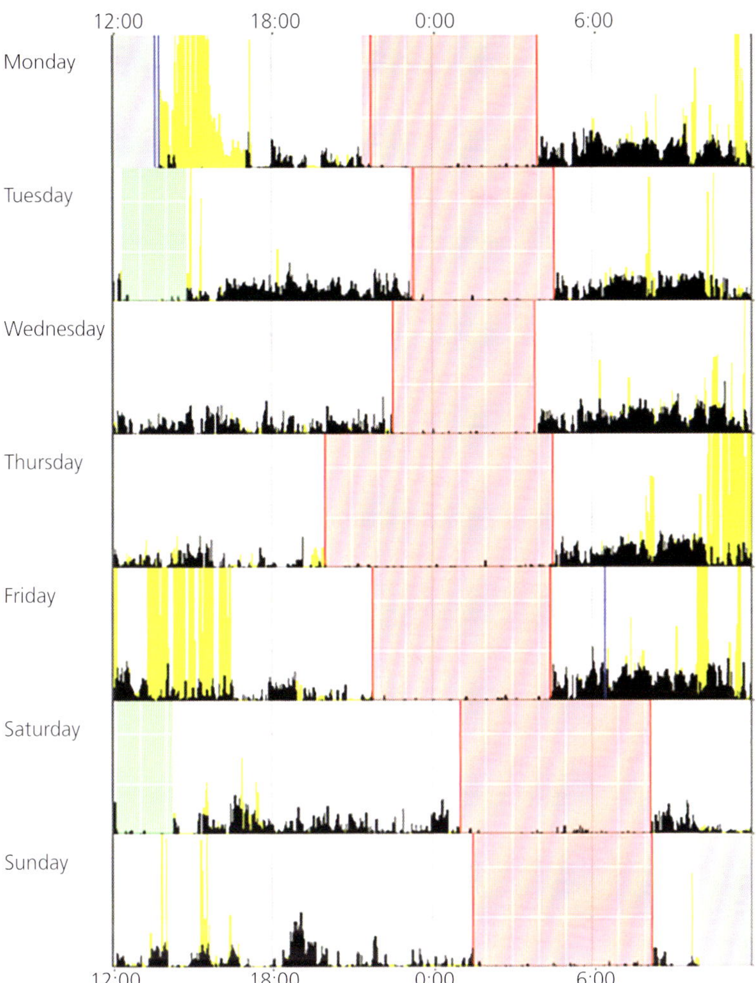

Figure 2.1 A 24-hour actogram with data from 1 week showing an irregular sleep–wake rhythm and sleep curtailment. Mean time in bed (pink) = 6.3 hours (range 5.32–6.32 hours); movement, black; daytime nap, green; light intensity, yellow; device not worn, gray.

awake while comfortably seated in a quiet room with a dim light. No activity or talking is allowed. The MWT consists of four 40-minute sessions performed at 2-hour intervals. Sleep onset is defined as the first period of more than 15 seconds of cumulative sleep in a 30-second time period. Sessions are terminated after 40 minutes if no sleep occurs or after sleep, defined as three consecutive periods of stage-1 sleep or one period of any other stage of sleep. A sleep technologist must be present to score sleep. The primary outcome measure is the mean sleep latency over the four sessions.

The Oxford Sleep Resistance test is a behavioral version of the MWT in which polysomnography is not applied. It follows the same schedule and participants are similarly comfortably seated. Instead of electroencephalic recording of sleep onset, participants are required to respond to a non-arousing visual stimulus. The participant's index finger is placed on a sensor. A light-emitting diode is positioned 1.2–1.8 m away at eye level in the frontal visual field. The light flashes regularly for 1 second every 3 seconds. Participants are instructed to remove their finger from the sensor for 1 second when the red light flashes. Sleep onset is defined as seven consecutive omissions, essentially non-responding to flashes. Similar to the MWT, a session is terminated at sleep onset or after 40 minutes of being awake. The primary outcome measure is the mean of the four sleep-onset latencies. The Oxford Sleep Resistance test has the advantage of not requiring the constant presence of a sleep technologist.

Objective tests for vigilance

The Sustained Attention to Response Task is a go/no-go test in which the no-go target appears unpredictably and rarely, and in which both accuracy and response speed, quantified as reaction time, are important.[6] It lasts 4 minutes and 19 seconds, and comprises the numbers 1–9 appearing 225 times in random order and at different sizes in a white font on a black computer screen. Participants have to respond to the appearance of each number by pressing a button while seated in a room that is dimly lit, except when the number is a 3, which occurs 25 times in total. Participants have to press the button before the next number appears and are instructed to give equal importance to accuracy and speed in performing the task. The primary outcome measure of the test is the total error score.

The psychomotor vigilance test is a simple reaction-time test. Participants are instructed to press a button as quickly as possible to stop a digital millisecond counter, which starts to scroll at variable intervals (interstimuli intervals: 2–10 seconds). The task requires continuous attention to detect the randomly occurring stimuli. Tests of varying duration are available but the best-validated duration is 10 minutes. Outcome measures vary between studies but the frequency of lapses, the average reaction time, and the average of the 10% slowest or fastest reaction times per session are frequently used.

Key points – clinical features and diagnosis

- EDS is not only characterized by daily episodes of an irrepressible need to sleep or daytime lapses into sleep, but often also by impaired sustained attention, automatic behavior, cognitive complaints and sometimes sleep inertia.
- It is important that EDS is separated from tiredness and fatigue, which are qualitatively different complaints.
- The most frequent cause of EDS is chronic sleep deprivation induced by sleep curtailment and/or a severely disturbed sleep–wake rhythm. OSA is the sleep disorder that most frequently causes EDS.
- Neither the characteristics of the EDS complaint, nor the results of polysomnographic recordings can reliably determine if EDS is behaviorally induced or caused by a disorder.
- Sleep registrations (including the MSLT) should be conducted if complaints remain after sleep extension and/or treatment of existing OSA. Ancillary investigations can focus on all aspects of EDS/ENS and it is best to use several approaches during the diagnostic process.

References

1. American Academy of Sleep Medicine. *International Classification of Sleep Disorders*, 3rd edn. American Academy of Sleep Medicine, 2014.
2. Lammers GJ, Bassetti CLA, Dolenc-Groselj L et al. Diagnosis of central disorders of hypersomnolence: a reappraisal by European experts. *Sleep Med Rev* 2020;52:101306.
3. Ruigt GSF, van Gerven J. The effects of medication on sleep and wakefulness. In: Overeem S, Reading P, eds. *Sleep Disorders in Neurology: A Practical Approach*, 2nd edn. Wiley-Blackwell, 2018:83–126.
4. Johns MW. A new method for measuring daytime sleepiness: the Epworth Sleepiness Scale. *Sleep* 1991;14:540–5.
5. Littner MR, Kushida C, Wise M et al. Practice parameters for clinical use of the multiple sleep latency test and the maintenance of wakefulness test. *Sleep* 2005;28:113–21.
6. Lammers GJ, van Schie M, van Dijk JG. Daytime tests for sleepiness and vigilance: indications, interpretations and pitfalls. In: Overeem S, Reading P, eds. *Sleep Disorders in Neurology: A Practical Approach*, 2nd edn. Wiley-Blackwell, 2018:31–46.

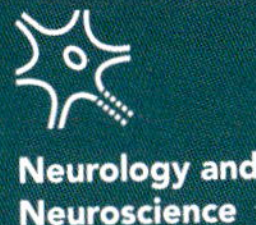

3 Management

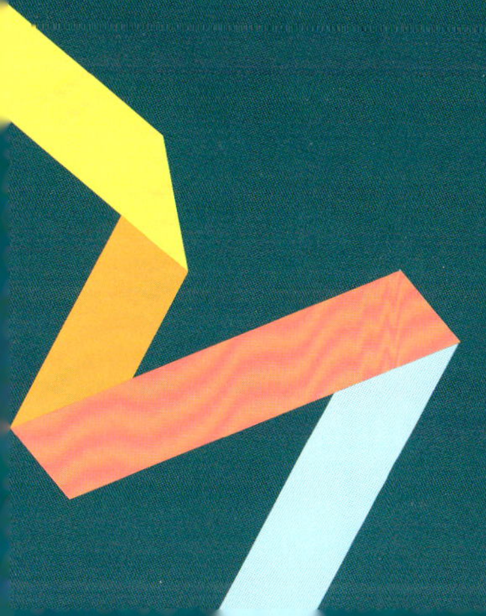

Management of EDS in patients with OSAS is an important issue, but best practice is not well defined because no evidence-based guidelines are available; as a result, there are uncertainties about the best treatment approaches in clinical practice. Guidance from the UK's National Institute for Health and Care Excellence outlines one approach that addresses the matter.[1]

Management of EDS in patients with OSAS generally requires a stepwise approach because the presentation and cause of the corresponding symptoms can vary, and may potentially require different treatment approaches (Figure 3.1).

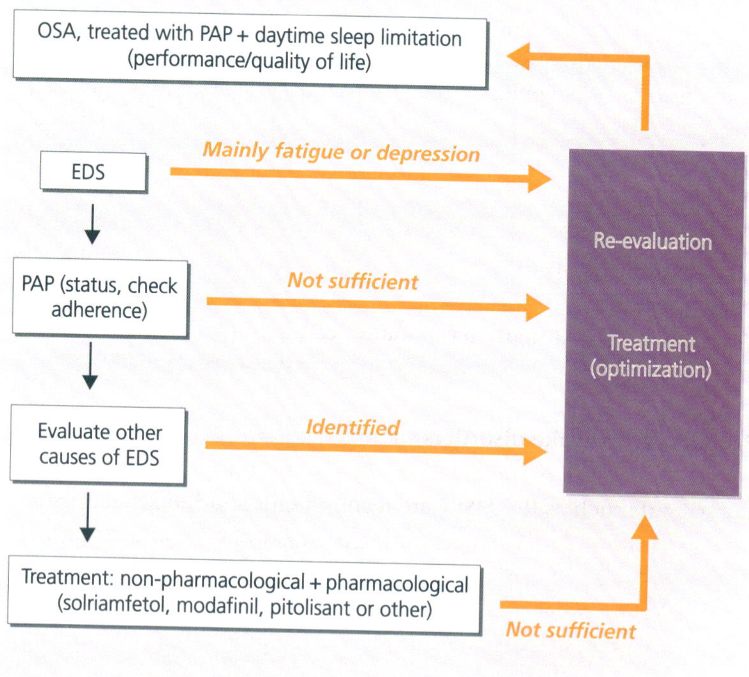

Figure 3.1 Treatment algorithm for patients with OSAS reporting EDS. PAP, positive airway pressure.

Considerations

In patients with OSAS, daytime symptoms, referred to as (residual) EDS, include a broad spectrum of disturbances, including tiredness, fatigue, cognitive deficit, loss of motivation, lethargy and EDS in the narrow sense, which reduce quality of life. Precise differentiation of the presented symptomatology can be made by clinical history taking (see Chapter 2), and sleep–wake examination – including polysomnography, MSLT, actigraphy and others – can add helpful objective information (see Figure 3.1).

Depression and fatigue. Patients describing symptoms of depression such as lethargy or apathy may benefit from antidepressive therapy. For patients reporting fatigue, treatment can be different from that for EDS; periods of rest during the day may be more important and useful than, for example, scheduled napping. They may also benefit from antidepressive pharmacological therapy in addition to stimulant therapy.

Sleep deprivation is one of the most frequent causes of EDS. Therapeutically, an extension of sleep duration, usually to at least 7 hours per night, is recommended. Sleep duration varies individually, particularly in younger patients; the necessary mean sleep duration may be 8 hours per night. Sleep diaries can help patients to achieve extended sleep duration and actigraphy may also be applied.

Primary sleep–wake disorders such as narcolepsy, also called central disorders of hypersomnolence (Table 3.1),[2] need to be considered and assessments such as the MSLT are recommended. If identified, specific treatments for primary hypersomnolence disorders should be applied.[3]

Non-pharmacological management

There are very limited data regarding non-pharmacological treatment approaches other than positive airway pressure (PAP) for EDS in patients with OSA. A regular sleep–wake pattern including enough sleep (>7 hours), regular physical exercise, weight reduction, not smoking, reducing alcohol consumption in the evening/night and scheduled napping (at least one short nap lasting approximately 15 minutes around noon) are likely to be beneficial (also see Chapter 4).[4]

TABLE 3.1

Primary sleep–wake disorders

- Narcolepsy (types 1 and 2)
- Idiopathic hypersomnia
- Kleine-Levin syndrome (periodic hypersomnia)
- Hypersomnia associated with a psychiatric or medical disorder, or due to a medication or substance

Adapted from American Academy of Sleep Medicine, 2014.[2]

Only patients describing EDS (see history taking), who regularly and successfully use PAP therapy, and for whom other causes of EDS have been excluded should be described as having 'EDS in OSA' or 'residual EDS in OSA'. The pathophysiology of EDS in OSA is still not well understood. OSA is common in middle-aged men with metabolic syndrome; however, it remains unclear whether OSA has a particular impact on EDS, or OSA and 'residual EDS' simply coexist ('residual EDS in OSA').[5]

Positive airway pressure is the first-line therapy for symptomatic moderate-to-severe OSA. PAP refers to all sleep apnea treatments that use a stream of compressed air to support the airway during sleep. PAP normalizes the AHI, suppresses nocturnal oxygen desaturations, decreases sleep fragmentation, and usually improves daytime sleepiness and fatigue.[4–8]

Patients with OSA treated with PAP who still suffer from EDS should first undergo polygraphic and/or polysomnographic PAP therapy re-evaluation.[7] Depending on the findings – particularly reduction of the AHI to less than 5 per hour, desaturation indices, and the existence and proportion of central apnea – optimization of CPAP levels or switching to another PAP mode (such as automatic PAP, bilevel PAP or adaptive servo ventilation) may be recommended. A change of mask may also be helpful. It is also important to consider the presence of obesity hypoventilation syndrome or comorbidity with chronic obstructive pulmonary disease, as hypercapnia can be present in both disorders and result in EDS.[9]

Because 15% of patients with OSA refuse to try PAP and 20–30% discontinue PAP therapy over time,[10] adherence is a major issue that needs to be considered in patients with OSA experiencing EDS. Major causes of non-adherence include the amount of noise made by pumps and machines not being very portable, but mainly include masks being uncomfortable, inconvenience, claustrophobia and sometimes cost. Another key aspect is PAP therapy failing to improve disturbed sleep and/or daytime symptoms, resulting in treatment discontinuation. Regular (>90% of the time) use of PAP therapy for a duration of at least 4 hours, but ideally 6 hours, per night is recommended.

Assessment of other factors related to EDS (see Chapter 2) should be addressed following a PAP efficacy and adherence review. If the EDS is likely to be due to an underlying medical or neurological disorder, management of the disorder should be considered first. Similarly, the taking of any medication that may result in EDS should be reviewed. One of the most frequent reasons for EDS is sleep deprivation, and clinical history taking, the use of sleep diaries and actigraphy can identify such disturbance.

Stimulation therapy and mandibular advancement. Limited data indicate that mandibular advancement devices (MADs) may improve EDS in patients with OSA.[11] The effectiveness of stimulation therapy (for example, of the hypoglossal nerve) is unknown.

Pharmacological management

For treatment of depressive symptoms and fatigue see 'Considerations' (page 31). In patients with 'residual EDS in OSA' (see page 32), different wake-promoting drugs are used in addition to non-pharmacological management approaches.[12] All treatments are symptomatic and are usually used as monotherapy (Table 3.2). Two drugs have been formally approved for the treatment of EDS in OSA in Europe, and three in the USA, and reimbursement of most drugs has not been established.

Several compounds have been studied and are used for the treatment of EDS in patients with narcolepsy or attention deficit

TABLE 3.2

Wake-promoting drugs

Drug (mechanism of action)	Efficacy (main results)	Frequent adverse events	Maximum dosage
Modafinil (dopaminergic)	Improved ESS and MWT	Headache	400 mg/day
Solriamfetol (dopaminergic and norepinephrinergic)	Improved ESS and MWT	Headache, nausea	150 mg/day
Pitolisant (histaminergic)	Improved ESS and fatigue	Headache, insomnia	36 mg/day

disorder, such as methylphenidate. It has been concluded that such drugs are likely to be useful for the improvement of EDS in patients with OSA, although no direct studies have been reported.

Modafinil was the first drug to be studied for effectiveness in the treatment of EDS in patients with OSA. Improvement in EDS measured by the ESS (from 14.2 to 9.6 points) and behavioral alertness, and reduced functional impairment have been reported with modafinil, up to 400 mg/day.[13] Another study reported an improvement of sleep latency of 2.8 minutes as measured by the MWT.[14] Modafinil is approved for use in the USA but not in Europe.

Solriamfetol is a selective dopamine and norepinephrine reuptake inhibitor. Several studies have shown efficacy regarding EDS. In the TONES 3 study,[15] a population of patients with OSA with EDS who were undergoing (two-thirds) or had undergone (one-third) sleep apnea treatment was studied. Solriamfetol was shown to significantly increase wakefulness according to the ESS and extend sleep latency according to the MWT (Figure 3.2). No differences in response were observed between subgroups of participants who were adherent or non-adherent to primary OSA therapy. Most adverse events were mild or moderate in severity, and included headache (10.1%), nausea (7.9%), decreased appetite (7.6%), anxiety (7.0%) and nasopharyngitis (5.1%).

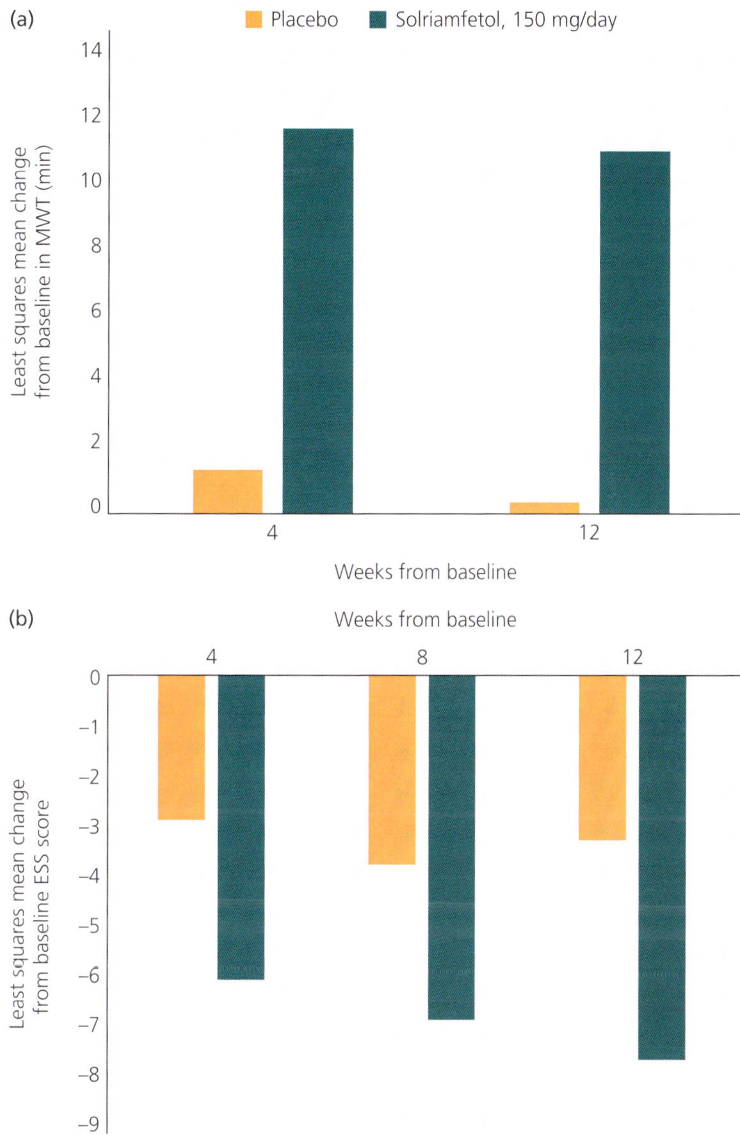

Figure 3.2 Changes in (a) MWT and (b) ESS from baseline over time with solriamfetol, 150 mg/day (n = 116) or placebo (n = 114). After 12 weeks, mean improvements of 11 minutes from baseline and –7.7 points on the ESS scale were documented with solriamfetol for MWT and ESS, respectively ($p < 0.0001$). Adapted from Schweitzer et al. 2019.[15]

Solriamfetol, up to 150 mg/day, has subsequently been approved by the US Food and Drug Administration and the European Medicines Agency (EMA) for the treatment of EDS in patients with OSA.[16]

Pitolisant is a selective histamine H3 receptor antagonist that increases histamine levels in the central nervous system. Since 2016, it has been used for the treatment of EDS and of cataplexy in patients with narcolepsy. The HAROSA II trial, which investigated patients with moderate-to-severe OSA who refused CPAP treatment, reported improvements in ESS (–3.3 points) (Figure 3.3) and Pichot fatigue scores with pitolisant, titrated up to 20 mg/day over 12 weeks, although MWT sleep latency values did not improve significantly. The most frequently reported adverse events were headache (8.5%), followed by insomnia, nausea and vertigo.[10] More recently, the HAROSA I trial reported significant differences between the placebo and pitolisant treatment groups for both ESS and MWT (as measured by the Oxford

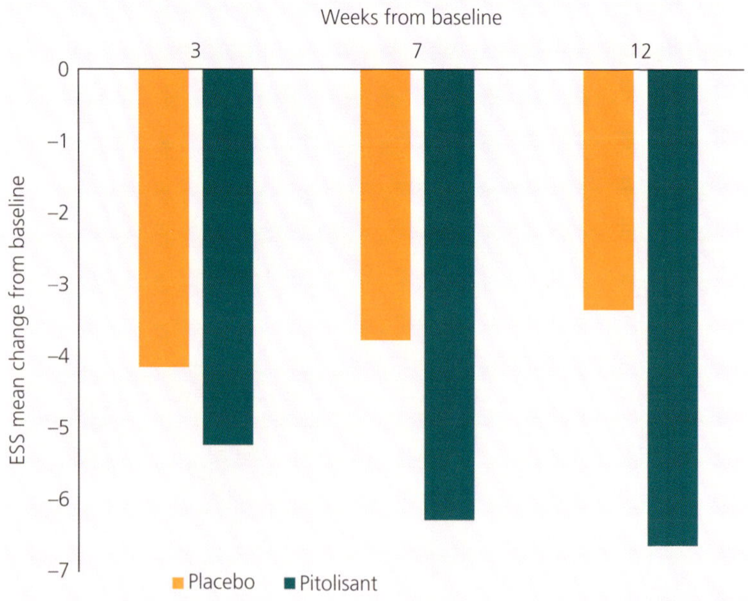

Figure 3.3 Changes in ESS score during treatment with pitolisant, titrated up to 20 mg/day over 12 weeks. An improvement of 6.6 points from baseline was reported. Adapted from Dauvilliers et al., 2020.[10]

Sleep Resistance Test) scores.[17] Pitolisant was recently approved for use by the EMA.

Special populations and situations

Treatment-resistant EDS. In some patients, EDS cannot be sufficiently improved by non-pharmacological and pharmacological treatment. In such cases, re-evaluation of other causes of EDS is recommended. If treatment with a pharmacological drug is not improving the EDS or cannot be continued because of adverse events, switching to another drug is necessary. Modafinil and solriamfetol are both dopaminergic stimulants, although solriamfetol is also norepinephrinergic, while pitolisant is histaminergic and is considered to be a wake-promoting drug. Thus, switching between the three may be helpful for treatment-resistant patients. Combination of a dopaminergic stimulant (for example, modafinil or solriamfetol) with a wake-promoting drug (for example, pitolisant) may be considered. Combination of dopaminergic stimulants is not recommended.

Cardiovascular comorbidities. OSA is most prevalent in middle-aged populations, particularly in men, and often coexists with metabolic syndrome. Such patients, and the elderly, often have cardiovascular disorders. Stimulants such as modafinil and solriamfetol often increase blood pressure, and the use of some drugs increases the risk of tachycardia and cardiac dysrhythmias; thus, the suitability of such stimulants for patients should be checked, particularly if they also have a cardiovascular disorder.

Beside potential cardiovascular side effects, some experts have expressed concern about prescribing stimulant or wake-promoting drugs to patients without non-pharmacological OSA treatment, and that patients may discontinue their treatment for OSA because their PAP or MAD treatment does not convincingly improve their quality of life when also treated with stimulants or wake-promoting drugs. Discontinuation of PAP and or MAD treatment may add to a patient's cardiovascular risk, although no data have been published to date that justify this concern.

Children. EDS in OSA in children after adequate treatment is very rare and other potential causes of EDS need to be evaluated carefully. Regarding management, non-pharmacological approaches should have priority and pharmacological treatment should only be applied in exceptional circumstances. No studies have evaluated the impact of stimulating drugs in this population to date.

Key points – management

- The diagnosis of residual EDS in patients with OSA is a process of exclusion; if applicable, other causes of EDS should be addressed and treated first.
- Management is purely symptomatic and includes the re-evaluation and optimization of PAP therapy, other non-pharmacological approaches and pharmacological treatment.
- After exclusion of sleep deprivation as a cause, data regarding non-pharmacological treatment approaches other than PAP for EDS in patients with OSA are limited.
- Achievement of a regular sleep–wake pattern including enough sleep (>7 hours), regular physical exercise, weight reduction, not smoking, reducing alcohol consumption in the evening/night and scheduled napping (at least one short nap lasting approximately 15 minutes around noon) are likely to be beneficial.
- Solriamfetol and pitolisant are approved for the treatment of EDS in OSA in Europe and the USA. Modafinil is approved in the USA but not in Europe.

References

1. National Institute for Health and Care Excellence. Obstructive sleep apnoea/hypopnoea syndrome and obesity hypoventilation syndrome in over 16s. NICE guideline [NG202]. 2021; www.nice.org.uk/guidance/ng202, last accessed 8 September 2021.
2. American Academy of Sleep Medicine. *International Classification of Sleep Disorders*, 3rd edn. American Academy of Sleep Medicine, 2014.
3. Bassetti CLA, Kallweit U, Vignatelli L et al. European guideline and expert statements on the management of narcolepsy in adults and children. *Eur J Neurol* 2021;28:2815–30.
4. Sánchez AI, Martínez P, Miró E et al. CPAP and behavioral therapies in patients with obstructive sleep apnea: effects on daytime sleepiness, mood, and cognitive function. *Sleep Med Rev* 2009;13:223–33.
5. Lammers GJ, Bassetti CLA, Dolenc-Groselj L et al. Diagnosis of central disorders of hypersomnolence: a reappraisal by European experts. *Sleep Med Rev* 2020;52:101306.
6. Chotinaiwattarakul W, O'Brien LM, Fan L, Chervin RD. Fatigue, tiredness, and lack of energy improve with treatment for OSA. *J Clin Sleep Med* 2009;5:222–7.
7. Foster SN, Hansen SL, Scalzitti NJ et al. Residual excessive daytime sleepiness in patients with obstructive sleep apnea treated with positive airway pressure therapy. *Sleep Breath* 2020;24:143–50.
8. Tomfohr LM, Ancoli-Israel S, Loredo JS, Dimsdale JE. Effects of continuous positive airway pressure on fatigue and sleepiness in patients with obstructive sleep apnea: data from a randomized controlled trial. *Sleep* 2011;34:121–6.
9. Castiglioni P, Lombardi C, Cortelli P, Parati G. Why excessive sleepiness may persist in OSA patients receiving adequate CPAP treatment. *Eur Respir J* 2012;39:226–7.
10. Dauvilliers Y, Verbraecken J, Partinen M et al. Pitolisant for daytime sleepiness in patients with obstructive sleep apnea who refuse continuous positive airway pressure treatment. A randomized trial. *Am J Respir Crit Care Med* 2020;201:1135–45.
11. Silva Gomes Ribeiro CV, Ribeiro-Sobrinho D, Muñoz Lora VRM et al. Association between mandibular advancement device therapy and reduction of excessive daytime sleepiness due to obstructive sleep apnea. *J Oral Rehabil* 2019;46:1031–5.

12. Sahni AS, Carlucci M, Malik M, Prasad B. Management of excessive sleepiness in patients with narcolepsy and OSA: current challenges and future prospects. *Nat Sci Sleep* 2019;11:241–52.
13. Dinges DF, Weaver TE. Effects of modafinil on sustained attention performance and quality of life in OSA patients with residual sleepiness while being treated with nCPAP. *Sleep Med* 2003;4:393–402.
14. Inoue Y, Miki M, Tabata T. Findings of the Maintenance of Wakefulness Test and its relationship with response to modafinil therapy for residual excessive daytime sleepiness in obstructive sleep apnea patients adequately treated with nasal continuous positive airway pressure. *Sleep Med* 2016;27–8:45–8.
15. Schweitzer PK, Rosenberg R, Zammit GK et al. Solriamfetol for excessive sleepiness in obstructive sleep apnea (TONES 3). A randomized controlled trial. *Am J Respir Crit Care Med* 2019;199:1421–31.
16. Schweitzer PK, Mayer G, Rosenberg R et al. Randomized controlled trial of solriamfetol for excessive daytime sleepiness in OSA: an analysis of subgroups adherent or nonadherent to OSA treatment. *Chest* 2021;160:307–18.
17. Pépin J-L, Georgiev O, Tiholov R et al. Pitolisant for residual excessive daytime sleepiness in OSA patients adhering to CPAP: a randomized trial. *Chest* 2021;159:1598–609.

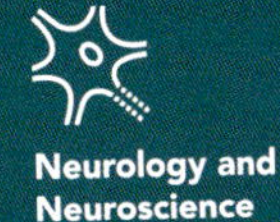

4 Patient impact and support

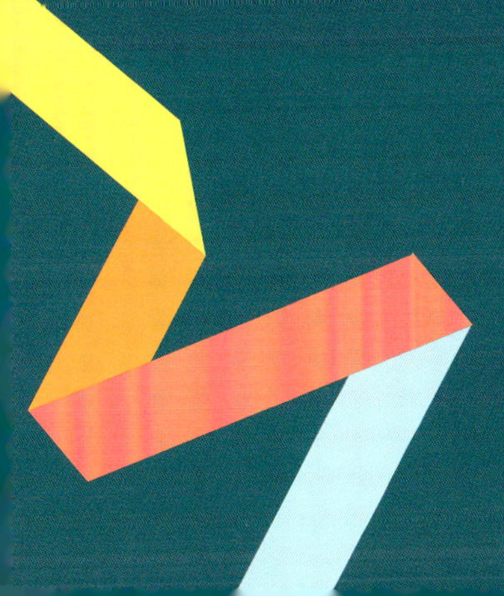

HEALTHCARE

With additional contribution from Kevin Ferrao, Faculty of Life Sciences and Medicine, King's College London, London, UK

Definitions

Seven major categories of sleep disorders are defined in the current ICSD-3 (Table 4.1).[1]

Sleep-related breathing disorders are characterized by disordered ventilation during sleep. Patients either experience decreasing levels of oxygen (hypoxia), increasing levels of carbon dioxide (hypercapnea), increased airway resistance (obstruction), cessation of respiratory drive (central apnea) or a mixture of the above.

OSA is a disorder in which a person repeatedly experiences obstruction of the upper airway while asleep, leading to diminished or absent airflow. The patient stops breathing and, eventually, arouses from sleep to overcome the upper airway obstruction, restore patency and rebreathe.[2] This repetitive pattern leads to sleep fragmentation and patients typically have complaints of EDS, and feel more tired and

TABLE 4.1

Sleep disorders, as defined by the ICSD-3

- Insomnia
- Sleep-related breathing disorders
  - Central sleep apnea syndromes
  - OSA disorders (the most common)
  - Sleep-related hypoventilation disorders
  - Sleep-related hypoxemia disorder
- Central disorders of hypersomnolence
- Circadian rhythm sleep–wake disorders
- Parasomnias
- Sleep-related movement disorders
- Other sleep disorders

Adapted from American Academy of Sleep Medicine, 2014.[1]

less refreshed the next day. When OSA is treated and normal breathing resumes, daytime symptoms such as EDS typically improve.

Effects of excessive daytime sleepiness

The causes of EDS can range from sleep disorders, sleep restriction, neurological and psychiatric conditions, and cardiovascular, metabolic or hematologic disorders, to the use of illicit/prescription drugs and poor sleep hygiene.[3]

EDS can negatively affect a person's work, social or family life and can have negative socioeconomic consequences, including psychological effects on the patient and their families and friends. Clinical research has highlighted the association between EDS and several mood disorders. Other important effects include sleepiness being involved in approximately 16% of road traffic accidents in England. It is also a risk factor when using heavy machinery.[4]

The effects of EDS emphasize its importance to primary care providers and patients. Ideally, EDS should improve when patients are treated for OSA. However, residual EDS can occur in a proportion of patients receiving treatment. Patient experiences of EDS may aid others who have similar symptoms through knowledge sharing and the development of support networks. As such, this chapter will primarily focus on the patient's experience and perspective of EDS, specifically for patients with OSA.

Benefits of good-quality sleep

The function of sleep is still not fully understood; however, as a mechanism that leaves human beings vulnerable to attack, it would not have been evolutionarily conserved if it was not important. A central role of sleep is to maintain our body in an optimized state, to enable it to 're-energize'; sleep aids recuperation from illness and injury, but also day-to-day maintenance such as memory formation, critical thinking and emotional, hormonal, immune, cardiovascular and metabolic regulation. Recent improved understanding of the glymphatic system underlines the importance of sleep in aiding the clearance of metabolic products from the central nervous system. These health benefits are the reverse of the effects caused by insufficient and fragmented sleep.

The effects of insufficient sleep

Insufficient sleep is defined as a curtailed sleep pattern that has persisted for at least 3 months, for most days of the week, along with the person complaining of sleepiness during the day.[1] This can become a problem when the individual's sleep cannot support adequate wakeful alertness, performance and health. Acute sleep deprivation is defined as no sleep or diminished total sleep time, usually lasting for 1–2 days. In contrast, chronic sleep insufficiency, also known as sleep restriction, occurs when an individual routinely sleeps less than the required amount for optimal functioning.[5] This can be voluntary or involuntary (for example, insomnia). Insufficient sleep can cause a variety of physical and mental dysfunctions, with some of the most important ones outlined below.

An irresistible urge to sleep during the day, often out of the control of the individual, most commonly occurs during a lack of physical activity, such as when driving.[5]

A decreased state of alertness is a common but dangerous effect of insufficient sleep. Normal alertness is when a person wakes up feeling refreshed and can go about their daily activities feeling alert without effort, even in boring or monotonous situations.[5] Many factors can cause decreased vigilance, one of the most common being alcohol consumption. To avoid fatal road traffic accidents, the law stipulates that people should not drive when they experience decreased states of alertness, no matter what the cause.

Decreased cognitive performance is the hallmark of sleep deprivation and can be directly linked to insufficient sleep. Research shows that sleep-deprived individuals have difficulty focusing and maintaining attention, recalling memories, and experience reduced strategic planning capacity and alertness.[3] These effects can contribute to poor school performance in sleep-deprived adolescents.[6]

Low mood, irritability and poor judgment have also been shown to be caused by insufficient sleep,[4] and increased anxiety is one of the most important consequences of sleep deprivation.[7] Irritability, moodiness and poor frustration tolerance are the most commonly reported symptoms in people experiencing sleep restriction.[8]

Increased cardiovascular morbidity has been linked with insufficient sleep.[5,8] The American Heart Association recognizes sleep restriction as increasing cardiometabolic risk including the risk of obesity, hypertension, type 2 diabetes and cardiovascular disease.[9]

Impaired immune function leading to weakened host defense against infectious disease is associated with chronic sleep loss.[8]

Obesity and metabolism. Chronic sleep restriction is thought to be a risk factor for obesity and impaired glucose metabolism.[5] A strong link has been reported between increased neck circumference (due to obesity) and the occurrence of OSA.[10]

Poor quality of life. Sleep-deprived individuals report that they do not have enough energy to participate in activities that they used to enjoy. Inappropriate naps and drowsiness cause embarrassment and friction at home, at work and during social events. Productivity decreases and contributes to diminished employability, while falling asleep at home may cause discontent in family life, including marital discord, contributing to low mood.[5]

Fitness to drive. Local legal guidelines vary between different sovereign countries (see Useful resources for European and British guidance). The UK's Driver and Vehicle Licensing Agency (DVLA) prioritises the symptom of EDS in individuals with OSA. Where EDS is absent, even if OSA is diagnosed or suspected, an individual may usually drive as normal. If EDS is present, then the individual must not drive until the symptom has resolved.[11]

Cultural perspectives

EDS is common worldwide; however, different cultures have varying views on EDS, with it being considered a variation of the norm in some societies. To further understand this, it is important to define the most common sleep patterns:[12]

- monophasic: sleeping once per day, at night-time only
- biphasic: sleeping twice per day, with a long sleep at night (6–7 hours) and a short nap during the day (up to 1 hour)
- polyphasic: multiple sleep periods per day, involving a short sleep at night with several short naps (20–30 minutes).

EDS is widely accepted in many cultures due to historic traditions (as seen in Spain as a result of the hot climate), society's expectation of normal work hours (as seen in Japan), interactions between modern culture and religion (as seen in many Arab Muslim countries), or even due to social pressure or expectation (Table 4.2).

As a result, EDS is not considered a problem or cause for concern in many cultures, one possible explanation being that EDS has arisen as a result of environmental and behavioral factors, as opposed to being due to a disorder, that can be treated. EDS may also be more acceptable given specific circumstances and therefore less likely to cause problems such as socioeconomic issues. An example that supports this is businesses in Spain and Italy (and many other hot countries) closing mid-afternoon to enable siestas and riposos, respectively.[13] In colder countries this would be expected to deter customers and would thus be less acceptable.

Lifestyle and sleep hygiene

There is little scientific evidence to support the recommendation of particular sleep durations because the need for sleep differs by individual and age. This is reflected in the National Sleep Foundation's recommendations, where recommended hours are reported next to 'may be appropriate' and 'not recommended' hours, signifying that individuals' sleep requirements vary.[14]

To maintain good sleep duration and quality, it is important that individuals adhere to a good sleep routine and sleep hygiene. Similarly, sufficient physical exercise and daylight exposure are important; these can help improve the induction and quality of sleep, and also help individuals avoid obesity and its associated detrimental effects on sleep, such as OSA. Limiting alcohol intake and avoiding caffeinated drinks, particularly late in the day, can help. In addition, a review of the sleep environment including light levels in the room, TV/modern media/ screen use in the evening or use of mobile phones in the bedroom, blinds on the windows to avoid light interference and nocturnal room

TABLE 4.2

Different cultural perspectives of EDS

Culture	Name	Sleep pattern	Description
Most industrialized and developed countries	N/A	Monophasic	Many workers and children sleep only once, at night
Spain and many Latin American countries	Siesta, meaning mid-afternoon break	Biphasic	Closely linked to Spanish culture, naps are usually taken between 2 and 5 PM in addition to a night-time sleep
Italy	Riposo, meaning mid-afternoon break	Biphasic	Naps are usually taken during the hottest time of the day
Japan	Inemuri, meaning being present while asleep	Mainly polyphasic	The intense work culture sees people taking naps wherever possible (park, library, daily commute etc.), which is seen as proof of hard work because night-time sleep has been sacrificed for productivity
Many Middle Eastern countries with large Muslim populations	N/A	Biphasic/ polyphasic	Muslims take one or more naps depending on their night-time sleep quality; the five obligatory prayer times per day coupled with modern lifestyles (technology, late night socialising etc.) lead some to go to sleep later and wake earlier for morning prayer
Many adolescents and university students	N/A	Biphasic/ polyphasic	Poor quality and little sleep can be attributed to social pressure, poor time management and part-time work, resulting in poor night-time sleep with naps during the day

N/A, not applicable.

temperature may be useful. Rules for good sleep hygiene recommended by the World Sleep Society are outlined in Table 4.3.[15]

Patient support

EDS arising from OSA may leave many patients troubled and concerned. Sleep medicine is a relatively young field and many primary care providers, especially those who do not work in sleep centers, may not recognise EDS and/or correctly identify the effects on an individual's quality of life, leaving many people with sleep disorders undiagnosed. Although public awareness of OSA has improved in recent years following several awareness campaigns, residual symptoms that may require additional therapeutic approaches have lacked attention; as a result, primary care providers and patients have limited awareness, and it can be difficult for patients with residual EDS to access support.

A first port of call for people to get help is to contact support groups or charities for patients with OSA. They act as advocates and can help in many ways. Patient support groups provide a link between patients

TABLE 4.3

Rules for good sleep hygiene

- Establish regular bed and waking times
- Adopt a healthier lifestyle (reduce or cut out alcohol, smoking, drugs etc.)
- Create a caffeine cut-off time
- Do not have a bedtime snack
- Consider your workout routine
- Use comfortable, inviting bedding
- Keep the bedroom well ventilated and at a comfortable temperature
- Block out distracting noise and as much light as possible
- Only use your bed for sleep and sexual activity (avoid use for work/general recreation)

Adapted from World Sleep Society, 2020.[15]

and primary care providers, aiding both sleep clinics and patients. They provide concerned patients with education, information leaflets and valuable contacts, with an emphasis on information that has been verified by clinicians. They also help to increase awareness by stressing the importance of OSA, treatment, and the negative effects of insufficient or fragmented sleep in primary care and governmental contexts, such as with driving license agencies.

While most countries have OSA support groups (see Useful resources for a selection), two internationally active English language charities supporting patients in person or remotely are Hope2Sleep and the Sleep Apnoea Trust (SAT) (Table 4.4). Both charities are patient-centered with hands-on help and provide relevant contacts for their patients; they advocate for better OSA awareness and recognition of associated issues, such as EDS, and they strongly support patients' rights, for example in the context of driving. Both charities also have 'expert patients' who have had special mandatory training to enable them to talk to patients empathically without jeopardising any confidential information, while acknowledging the limitations of their guidance. Expert patients have been diagnosed with OSA themselves and, as a result, they are well prepared to listen to and understand the worries of people with OSA, putting them in a strategic position to offer aid. Access to other patients with similar experiences and information about CPAP therapy, mask fitting, social and financial support, driving and access to reputable clinicians for alternative treatment are the most common requests received.

TABLE 4.4

Support offered by SAT and Hope2Sleep

- Offer general support and legal information regarding OSA via website, newsletters, telephone, email, webinars, conferences and open days, and independent and externally approved health plans, including weight-loss advice for overweight and obese patients
- Host public events
- Advocate for the rights of patients with OSA (for example, with the DVLA)
- Organize and maintain support groups for patients to connect with each other
- Raise awareness of the importance of recognising OSA in primary care
- Support patient sleep clinics
- Collaborate with clinical academic and public health partners

Key points – patient impact and support

- EDS is not always a manifestation of an underlying sleep disorder.
- The most common sleep-related breathing disorder is OSA.
- Perception of EDS differs widely. However, EDS is often associated with significant adverse health impact.
- Sleep hygiene is important to promote good quality sleep in sufficient quantity.
- Patient support groups provide important help to those with underlying sleep disorders regarding their associated adverse health and social outcomes.

References

1. American Academy of Sleep Medicine. *International Classification of Sleep Disorders*, 3rd edn. American Academy of Sleep Medicine, 2014.
2. Park JG, Ramar K, Olson EJ. Updates on definition, consequences, and management of obstructive sleep apnea. *Mayo Clin Proc* 2011;86:549–55.
3. Bittencourt LR, Silva RS, Santos RF et al. Excessive daytime sleepiness. *Braz J Psychiatry* 2005;27:16–21.
4. Ohayon MM, Caulet M, Philip P et al. How sleep and mental disorders are related to complaints of daytime sleepiness. *Arch Intern Med* 1997;157:2645–52.
5. Cirelli C, Benca R, Eichler AF. *Insufficient Sleep: Definition, Epidemiology, and Adverse Outcomes*, 2021. www.uptodate.com/contents/insufficient-sleep-definition-epidemiology-and-adverse-outcomes, last accessed 8 September 2021.
6. Millman RP, Working Group on Sleepiness in Adolescents/Young Adults; AAP Committee on Adolescence. Excessive sleepiness in adolescents and young adults: causes, consequences, and treatment strategies. *Pediatrics* 2005;115:1774–86.
7. Pires GN, Bezerra AG, Tufik S, Andersen ML. Effects of acute sleep deprivation on state anxiety levels: a systematic review and meta-analysis. *Sleep Med* 2016;24:109–18.
8. Chattu VK, Manzar MD, Kumary S et al. The global problem of insufficient sleep and its serious public health implications. *Healthcare (Basel)* 2018;7:1.
9. St-Onge MP, Grandner MA, Brown D et al. Sleep duration and quality: impact on lifestyle behaviors and cardiometabolic health: a scientific statement from the American Heart Association. *Circulation* 2016;134:e367–86.
10. Reed K, Pengo MF, Steier J. Screening for sleep-disordered breathing in a bariatric population. *J Thorac Dis* 2016;8:268–75.
11. GOV.UK. *Miscellaneous Conditions: Assessing Fitness to Drive*, 2021. www.gov.uk/guidance/miscellaneous-conditions-assessing-fitness-to-drive, last accessed 11 May 2021.
12. Al-Abri MA, Al Lawati I, Zadjali F, Ganguly S. Sleep patterns and quality in Omani adults. *Nat Sci Sleep* 2020;12:231–7.

13. Deshong A. *How the World Naps*, 2021. www.sleep.org/napping-around-the-world/, last accessed 11 May 2021.
14. Hirshkowitz M, Whiton K, Albert SM et al. National Sleep Foundation's sleep time duration recommendations: methodology and results summary. *Sleep Health* 2015;1:40–3.
15. World Sleep Society. *10 Tips for Better Sleep Graphic*, 2020. https://worldsleepday.org/usetoolkit/resources/10-tips-for-better-sleep-graphic, last accessed 11 May 2021.

Useful resources

Professional societies

American Sleep Apnea Association (ASAA)
www.sleepapnea.org

American Sleep Association
www.sleepassociation.org

American Thoracic Society
Sleep Fragments
www.thoracic.org/professionals/clinical-resources/sleep/sleep-fragments/

British Sleep Society
www.sleepsociety.org.uk

European Sleep Research Society
https://esrs.eu

World Sleep Society
https://worldsleepsociety.org

Patient charities

Hope2Sleep
www.hope2sleep.co.uk

Sleep Apnoea Trust
https://sleep-apnoea-trust.org

Sleep Foundation
www.sleepfoundation.org

Guidance on driving

British Thoracic Society
Position Statement on Driving with OSA
https://sleep-apnoea-trust.org/wp-content/uploads/2020/08/BTS-Position-Statement-on-Driving-Obstructive-Sleep-Apnoea-OSA-2018.pdf

Driver & Vehicle Licensing Agency
www.gov.uk/government/publications/tiredness-can-kill-advice-for-drivers

European Respiratory Society
Statement on sleep apnea, sleepiness and driving
https://erj.ersjournals.com/content/erj/early/2020/09/28/13993003.01272-2020.full.pdf

Appendix: about the authors

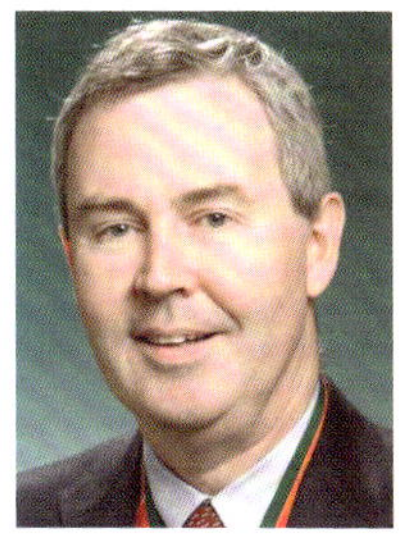

Walter T McNicholas MD FRCPI FERS is Consultant in Respiratory and Sleep Medicine at St. Vincent's Hospital Group, Dublin, and Newman Clinical Research Professor at University College Dublin, Ireland. He has published over 250 research papers in international peer-reviewed journals and is past President of both the European Sleep Research Society and the European Respiratory Society. He chaired a Working Group of the European Commission on Sleep Apnoea and Driving between 2012 and 2014, which led to an EU Directive on the topic that is now in force throughout Europe.

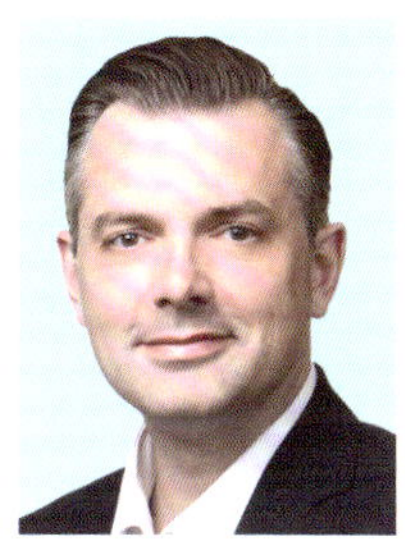

Ulf Kallweit MD FEAN is Associate Professor of Neurology at the University of Witten/Herdecke, Germany, and Head of the Center for Narcolepsy/Hypersomnias and the division of clinical sleep and neuroimmunology Research Professor at the Stanford Sleep Epidemiology Research Center, USA. His work focuses on the clinical aspects and management of narcolepsy and hypersomnolence disorders. He is Chair of both the Educational Committee of the European Narcolepsy Network and the Sleep Disorders Panel of the European Academy of Neurology, and recipient of the Nakano Citation (2019), the Research Prize in Neurosciences, Pfizer Foundation (2020) and first prize for Research in Neurodegenerative Diseases from the Franco Regli Foundation (2021). He was appointed Field Editor of the journal *Sleep Medicine* in 2021 and is Associated Editor of *Sleep Epidemiology*.

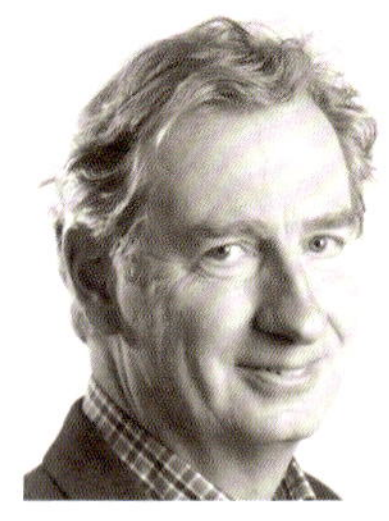

Gert Jan Lammers MD PhD FEAN is Professor of Neurology, Leiden University Medical Center and Medical Director of Sleep-Wake Center SEIN, The Netherlands. His main interests are central disorders of hypersomnolence, particularly narcolepsy, with diagnostic criteria, pathophysiology and expressions of impaired vigilance his main focus. He is past President and co-founder of the European Narcolepsy Network and the current Chair of the Dutch Sleep Medicine Society. He is much involved in education in sleep medicine and has published extensively (more than 180 PubMed-cited papers and numerous book chapters).

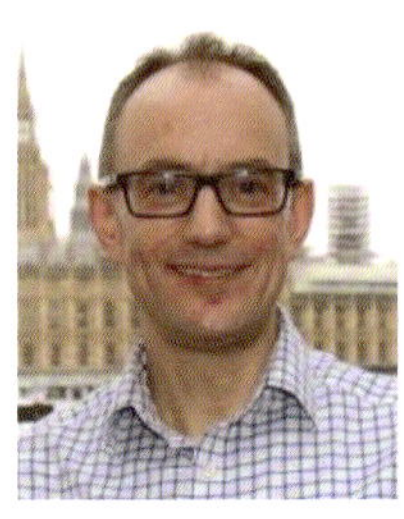

Joerg Steier MD PhD FRCP is Consultant at Guy's and St Thomas' NHS Foundation Trust in the Lane Fox Unit, a tertiary service for weaning and non-invasive ventilation, and the British Sleep Society-accredited Sleep Disorders Centre of King's Health Partners. He was awarded the chair of Respiratory and Sleep Medicine at King's College London. He is currently President of the British Sleep Society and a member of its executive committee, and a task force member of the European Respiratory Society.
His work in the field of respiratory and sleep physiology has evolved into collaborations across six continents.

INDEX